Isabella Altamirano
Elías Dubón
Alexander Jacomino

Biopower and Public Health

Isabella Altamirano
Elías Dubón
Alexander Jacomino

Biopower and Public Health

Biopower and Public Health Management

ScienciaScripts

Imprint

Any brand names and product names mentioned in this book are subject to trademark, brand or patent protection and are trademarks or registered trademarks of their respective holders. The use of brand names, product names, common names, trade names, product descriptions etc. even without a particular marking in this work is in no way to be construed to mean that such names may be regarded as unrestricted in respect of trademark and brand protection legislation and could thus be used by anyone.

Cover image: www.ingimage.com

This book is a translation from the original published under ISBN 978-613-9-46839-3.

Publisher:
Sciencia Scripts
is a trademark of
Dodo Books Indian Ocean Ltd. and OmniScriptum S.R.L publishing group

120 High Road, East Finchley, London, N2 9ED, United Kingdom
Str. Armeneasca 28/1, office 1, Chisinau MD-2012, Republic of Moldova, Europe
Managing Directors: Ieva Konstantinova, Victoria Ursu
info@omniscriptum.com

ISBN: 978-620-8-50882-1

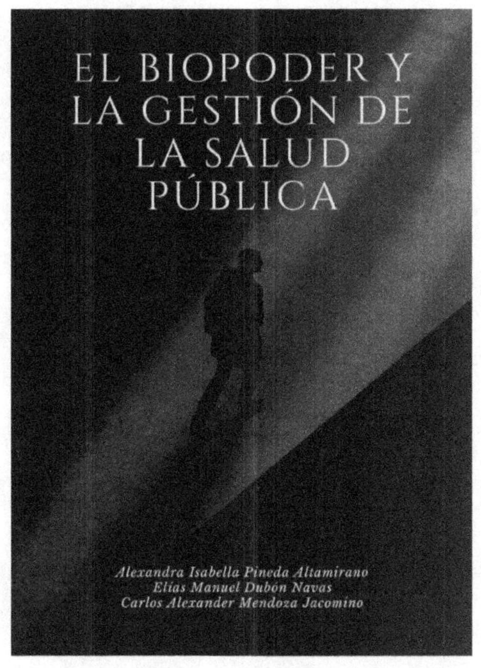

BIOPOWER AND PUBLIC HEALTH MANAGEMENT

TABLE OF CONTENTS

FOREWORD

In recent decades, humanity has witnessed significant advances in public health, from the eradication of diseases to the development of technologies capable of monitoring and predicting epidemic outbreaks. However, these advances have been accompanied by ethical and political challenges that question the limits of state intervention in people's lives. The COVID-19 pandemic, for example, not only tested health systems around the world, but also reignited debates about surveillance, individual autonomy and the power of the state in times of health crisis.In this context, the concept of biopower, developed by the philosopher Michel Foucault, emerges as a crucial tool for analysing the dynamics between power, health and life. Biopower refers to the set of practices through which authorities regulate the biological life of the population, using public health as a means of exercising control and managing risks. While this power is essential to protect communities, it also raises fundamental questions: to what extent can the state intervene in the lives of individuals? What happens when health policies affect rights such as privacy, freedom or autonomy? And, above all, how can we ensure that biopower is exercised fairly and equitably?This book delves into these questions, offering an in-depth and accessible reflection on how biopower influences public health management. With a clear and structured approach, the book covers the theoretical foundations of biopower, its practical application in pandemic and vaccination contexts, the associated ethical dilemmas, and the impact of new technologies on health surveillance. It also addresses future perspectives, considering the role of biopower in the face of global challenges such as climate change and globalisation.The reader will find here an analysis that is not only relevant for academics or health professionals, but also for anyone interested in understanding how decisions that affect their lives and well-being are made. In a world where health crises are becoming increasingly frequent, it is crucial to foster an informed and critical citizenry that actively

INTRODUCTION

Public health is one of the fundamental pillars for the development and well-being of any society. Throughout history, states have played a crucial role in protecting and promoting the health of their citizens, implementing various strategies to control diseases, improve access to health services and promote healthy behaviours. However, in the exercise of this power, there is a complex intersection between collective well-being and individual autonomy. This concept of state intervention in the health of the population, defined by Michel Foucault as "biopower", has become a focus of analysis for understanding how people's lives are managed and regulated in the name of public health.

The term biopower refers to a set of techniques and practices through which the state regulates and monitors the lives of its citizens in order to maintain the health of society as a whole. This regulation ranges from the implementation of vaccination campaigns and promotion of healthy habits, to the imposition of quarantines and mobility restrictions in health emergencies. Through biopower, governments have the ability to influence individuals' decisions about their own bodies and health, a power that is necessary to contain and mitigate health threats, but which also raises ethical questions about the limits of state intervention and respect for individual rights.

The COVID-19 pandemic has highlighted the importance and complexities of biopower in public health management. Measures such as containment, contact tracing and mandatory vaccination have been implemented by governments around the world to protect populations. However, these policies have also triggered intense debates about personal autonomy, privacy and surveillance. In this context, it is crucial to reflect on how biopower can be exercised ethically and equitably, ensuring collective well-being without transgressing individual rights. This book addresses the application of the concept of biopower in public health, with a particular focus on the ethical, technological and human rights challenges that emerge in health crisis situations. Through detailed analysis, we explore how biopower influences health policy, how new digital technologies expand the capacity to monitor and monitor health, and how biopower can be used as a tool to monitor and monitor the health of the population. and control, and what are the ethical limits of these practices in a context of individual rights. The aim of this book is to provide a comprehensive overview of the implications of biopower in public health, to offer tools for reflection and analysis that enable readers to understand the complex dynamics between state authority, health protection and respect for autonomy. The book is structured in eight chapters, organised in such a way that the reader is progressively introduced to the theoretical aspects of biopower. The first chapters define the concept of biopower and examine its application in public health policy, from a historical approach to its role in modernity. It then delves into the ethical dilemmas and human rights that arise in the practice of biopower, as well as the impact of new technologies on health control and surveillance. Finally, the last chapters explore the implications of biopower in a globalised context and the future challenges facing public health in the context of climate change and technological progress. Throughout this analysis, we seek to highlight the importance of responsible and balanced management of biopower in public health. Only through transparent and ethical governance can this power be used to promote well-being without compromising the freedom and dignity of individuals. This book, aimed at students, health professionals, academics and anyone interested in understanding the foundations and challenges of modern public health, offers a space for reflection on how to build healthy and just societies in an increasingly complex world.

CHAPTER 1

ORIGINS AND THEORY OF BIOPOWER

Introduction to the concept of biopower

Foucault defines biopower as the set of mechanisms by which power attempts to optimise the lives and bodies of individuals and populations. In contrast to sovereign power, which was exercised through the punishment or elimination of life, biopower focuses on managing life through strategies of regulation. Furthermore, it is important to consider how biopower has been influenced by social and political changes. Globalisation and technological advancement have transformed the dynamics of power, enabling new forms of control through data and digital surveillance. Biopower has emerged as a crucial concept for understanding the dynamics of power in our contemporary society and refers to the way in which political and social institutions regulate and manage the lives of individuals and populations. For Foucault biopower focuses on life, on the care of life, on the management of life, this perspective leads us to consider how power manifests itself not only through repression, but also through the optimisation and control of human existence. Biopower differs from traditional forms of power, which are based on coercion and domination. Instead of focusing on prohibition, biopower is concerned with the regulation and management of life. In this sense, it can be understood as a power that is exercised over people's bodies and health, where governments and institutions seeking to influence aspects such as birth rates, public health and social welfare has led to a reconfiguration of power relations, where the management of everyday life becomes a priority. As societies have evolved, biopower has taken on new dimensions. In contemporary contexts, we see how technologies, health policies and social norms intertwine to form a web of control that affects the population. As Agamben (2024) points out, biopower produces a new relationship between life and power, which implies that life itself becomes an object of regulation and management. This phenomenon has given rise to a wide-ranging debate about individual freedom, ethics and social responsibility. The concept of biopower, therefore, invites reflection on the role of the state and other institutions in the lives of citizens. It is crucial to understand that while biopower seeks to promote well-being and health, it can also give rise to practices of control and surveillance that limit individual autonomy. This raises questions about the balance between care for life and respect for personal freedom. Exploring these tensions is essential for a critical understanding of biopolitics today.

Michel Foucault and biopolitics

Foucault introduces biopolitics as a way of managing life at the level of populations. This form of power focuses on health, sexuality and reproduction, and is a tool of state control that seeks to maximise the capacity of the state to control the population. and the well-being of society.

In his work "History of Sexuality" Foucault explains how from the eighteenth century onwards, power has been oriented towards life, transforming the relationship between the individual and the state, power has become more productive than repressive; thus implying that, rather than simply imposing restrictions, power seeks to create and regulate conditions of life (Campos, 2010).

Biopolitics focuses on the strategies used by governments to manage the health, birth rate and well-being of the population. Foucault notes that this form of power manifests itself in institutions such as hospitals, schools and prisons, where practices are implemented that seek to optimise people's lives. This management of life is not neutral, it is influenced by ideologies and values that can perpetuate inequalities and exclusions. This trend is closely related to the rise of capitalism and modernity. In this context, control over life becomes a crucial aspect of economic production. As Oñate (2012) mentions, biopolitics becomes a regulatory mechanism that seeks to maximise the productivity of the population. This intersection between power, economy and life highlights the complexity of social relations in modernity. Foucault's analysis also raises important ethical questions. By focusing on life as an object of management, there is risk of dehumanising individuals, treating them mere resources within a system. It is therefore essential to question how these biopolitical practices are implemented and what implications they have for people's autonomy and dignity. Foucault's work invites us to reflect on the responsibility of institutions in shaping human lives.

Biopower in modernity and the management of life

Foucault argues that since the eighteenth century, institutions began to focus not only on political sovereignty, but also on the management of life itself, implying a shift in the paradigm of power. This approach focuses on power over bodies and populations, where the state takes an active role in promoting health and well-being. Since that date, biopower has become entrenched in public health systems, where disease control, hygiene and birth control policies are central. Over time, these policies have been integrated into government structures to regulate human life and encourage the "improvement" of populations. In modernity, this concept has manifested itself in diverse and complex ways, especially in the realm of health policy and social control. State institutions have adopted approaches that seek to optimise the lives of the population, but have also been responsible for practices of exclusion and marginalisation. As Esposito (2012) puts it, biopower is presented as a form of power that manages both life and death, revealing the ambivalence inherent in this concept.

Education has also been influenced by biopower, as educational institutions play a crucial role in shaping individuals to conform to social and economic norms. As García and González (2015) point out, modern education seeks not only to transmit knowledge, but also to shape behaviours and attitudes that align with the interests of the state. This function of education highlights how biopower infiltrates all spheres of social life, regulating not only health, but also ways of being and acting in society. It is important to consider the ethical and political implications of biopower in modernity. As institutions seek to manage people's lives, there is a need for a critical analysis that questions the dynamics of power and control. Biopolitics, therefore, should not only be seen as an instrument of management, but also as a field of resistance and transformation.

CHAPTER 2

PUBLIC HEALTH AND THE STATE'S ROLE IN LIFE MANAGEMENT

Definition of public health and its evolution

Public health is the discipline that focuses on disease prevention, health promotion and life extension through organised efforts by society. It has evolved from the simple eradication of diseases to the complex risk management and wellbeing. According to Muñoz (2000) the essential functions of public health include not only disease prevention, but also equitable access to health services. This implies that the state must adopt a proactive approach to address social determinants of health such as poverty, education and access to basic services.

The evolution of public health has been marked by different paradigms throughout history. From its origins in rudimentary hygiene and sanitation practices in ancient civilisations, to the development of more complex systems in the 20th century, public health has been adapting to the changing needs of populations (González, 2018). In this sense, the 19th century was a crucial period when more systematic health policies began to be implemented, driven by urban growth and epidemics affecting cities.

In 1946, the World Health Organisation WHO defined health as a state of complete physical, mental and social well-being, which significantly broadened the concept beyond the mere absence of disease (WHO, 1946). This contemporary definition underlines the importance of the social and environmental context in which a person lives. Modern public health focuses not only on medical interventions, but also on determinants such as education, access to basic services and socio-economic conditions.

Public health has also evolved to include intersectoral approaches that recognise that many factors influence health. For example, access to adequate housing, education and employment are essential for positive health outcomes (Crawford, 2006).

11

The role of the state in the health of the population

The state takes a central role in public health through policy and regulation. With the adoption of biopower, the state assumes responsibility for managing health resources and ensuring the wellbeing of its population, investing in medical infrastructure, preventive campaigns and disease control programmes. The right to health is an essential component of public policy that reflects the exercise of biopower. The World Health Organisation WHO (2017) defines health not only as the absence of disease, but as complete state of physical, mental and social well-being. This implies that public policies should go beyond medical treatment and include social interventions that promote a healthy environment. In this sense, biopower is manifested when the state regulates aspects such as food, housing and education to improve the overall health of the population.

The state has the capacity to implement laws and regulations that directly impact on the social determinants of health. For example, policies related to environmental sanitation, tobacco control or promotion of physical activities are clear examples of the role of the state in influencing healthy behaviours (López, 2014). These actions are essential to prevent diseases and promote a healthy environment for all citizens.

It is important for the state to coordinate efforts across different sectors to address complex health-related problems. Collaboration between ministries, non-governmental organisations and communities is vital to implement effective programmes that respond to local needs, which is why this intersectoral approach allows for a more comprehensive response to health challenges.

Adequate financing is another critical aspect of the state's role. Investment in health infrastructure and preventive programmes is essential to ensure an efficient and accessible health system; however, resources are often limited, posing significant challenges for governments to prioritise interventions that maximise the benefits to the population.

Legislation and public policies for health

Public health laws and government policies are essential tools of biopower. These policies range from the regulation of hygiene to the implementation of vaccination campaigns, setting the direction of the state intervention in the lives of citizens.

Legislation is a key component of public health management. Laws establish a normative framework that guides the actions of the state and defines the rights and responsibilities of both government and citizens with respect to health. For example, the General Health Law in Nicaragua establishes fundamental principles on the right to enjoy and preserve health (Asamblea Nacional de Nicaragua, 2007). This law regulates actions related to health promotion, prevention and recovery. Public policies are the tools through which these laws are implemented. Through well-designed policies, governments can address specific problems such as infectious or chronic diseases, thus ensuring an adequate response to health needs, as effective policy formulation and implementation requires constant analysis of their impact on the population.It is essential that public policies are inclusive and participatory. Citizen participation allows policies to truly reflect the needs and priorities of communities, which is why it is necessary to foster a culture of participation where citizens can be empowered to demand better health conditions and greater attention from the state. However, there are significant implementation challenges. Lack of financial or human resources can severely limit efforts to translate effective policies into concrete actions. An essential factor is to continuously evaluate these policies to ensure that they are meeting their objectives and adjust them as necessary.

CHAPTER 3

BIOPOWER AND SOCIAL CONTROL IN PUBLIC HEALTH

Monitoring instruments in public health

Control instruments include medical registries, epidemiological monitoring and vaccination campaigns. Through , the state establishes a surveillance system that allows it to respond to public health threats. Foucault points out that social control is exercised through rules and regulations that seek to shape behaviours considered healthy. For example, anti-smoking campaigns or programmes to promote healthy lifestyles reflect this dynamic.

Strategies used to exert this control include both incentives and sanctions. The promotion of healthy habits can be accompanied by restrictive policies that limit behaviours considered harmful to public health (Rosenberg and Kahn, 2011). However, these measures may generate ethical debates about the extent to which it is acceptable for the state to intervene in personal choices.

Action in public health is determined by two major circuits, that of information and that of decisions or that of data generation and use. The first focuses on defining the problem, selecting the information priorities needed to tackle it and collecting data (from where, from whom and how systematically). The analysis of the data and their interpretation will be the final elements to be able to draw up reports and specific recommendations that will go to the health authority, in our case at the regional level (if it is a regional problem) or at the national level if an intervention is required at the State level.

The use of information technologies to improve health management allows for more efficient tracking of health data, facilitating communication between different levels of the health system. This not only improves the response to health emergencies, but also optimises the use of resources by allowing a more precise allocation according to the needs detected.

Biopower in disease control infectious

Infectious diseases represent a threat that justifies the exercise of biopower. To minimise their spread, the state regulates the behaviour of citizens, controlling movement, imposing health measures and promoting vaccination. The management of biopower also implies a normalisation of social behaviour with regard to health. Preventive campaigns not only inform about risks, but also shape attitudes towards practices considered healthy or unhealthy. This process can lead to an internalisation by the individual, who begins to regulate his or her own behaviour as dictated by social norms imposed from above. Thus, biopower acts not only as a coercive mechanism, but also as a normative model that seeks to create a healthy population from an economic and political perspective.

Within the field of infectious diseases, some diseases in particular have an important impact on public health and generate significant pockets of disability, such as HIV infection, hepatitis and influenza. HIV infection has evolved very favourably thanks to new treatments, considerably increasing survival and quality of life. However, there is evidence of a more unfavourable evolution co-infections, such as hepatitis C. There are also increases in incidence and disability related to other causes common to the general population. As a consequence of survival, the prevalence of people alive and infected with HIV is steadily increasing, so the burden of disease and disability, as well as the labour and social cost, is rising. It would be interesting to establish lines of collaboration to assess the impact of this pathology on disability and invalidity.

It is important to consider how biopower is intertwined with the pharmaceutical and biotechnology industries. These industries operate within the biopower framework by developing treatments and vaccines that are essential for the control of infectious diseases. However, this also raises questions about the ethics behind equitable access to these products and how commercial decisions can influence health-related public policy.

Surveillance systems and preventive medicine

Lonsurveillance systems, such as immunisation registries and health databases, allow governments to collect information on the health of the population and are a key resource for preventing outbreaks. The term "surveillance" refers to a state of alertness and appropriate response to an individual's health by service providers in health care institutions, which requires systematic, decision-oriented observations regarding concrete measures to be implemented for prevention, medical care and rehabilitation of health. However, the term "health surveillance" or public health surveillance is currently used to refer to the state of health of the population, which involves the systematic search for information, its analysis and interpretation on the behaviour of health events in the population, the risk factors and determinants that condition them, in order to participate in the decision-making process aimed at improving the health of the population concerned. This definition implies and determines that the final link in the surveillance chain is the use of data and information in the promotion of health, prevention and control of diseases and their risk factors. It confirms something that is essential in the process: surveillance without immediate analysis and without alternative and timely proposals for action to correct identified deviations or contribute to them, is not surveillance and loses ownership as an essential function within the practice of public health.

Surveillance is information for action, it is a necessary and strategic component for both the development and sustainability of health systems and services; , it is the "cornerstone" of public health practice and an essential function, according to PAHO, from which strategic actions are derived that are necessary to contribute to the achievement of its central objective, which is also the purpose of public health: to improve the health of populations (Rodríguez, 2014).

The performance of health services and the satisfaction of users and service providers in the context of the influence of the determinants identified and studied in the different regions, contribute substantially to the establishment priorities and objectives. for action at different levels of the health system, contributes with its timely information to COUNTRIES OR REGIONS TO PREVENT AND ORGANISE THEIR RESPONSES TO EPIDEMIC SITUATIONS OF DISEASES OR DISASTERS AND IN THE PROMOTION OF HEALTH AND PREVENTION OF CHRONIC DISEASES. APPROPRIATE AND TIMELY DECISIONS CAN SAVE HUMAN LIVES AND PRESERVE YEARS OF LIFE WITHOUT DISABILITY, AS WELL AS CONTRIBUTE TO REDUCING THE COSTS OF DEALING WITH THE HEALTH PROBLEM IN QUESTION, THUS POSITIVELY INFLUENCING THE REDUCTION OF ITS SOCIAL AND ECONOMIC IMPACT.

CHAPTER 4

BIOPOWER IN CONTEXTS OF PANDEMIC

The COVID-19 pandemic: a contemporary case

The COVID-19 pandemic has been a global phenomenon that has highlighted the dynamics of biopower in public health management. This concept, developed by Michel Foucault, refers to the ways in which governments exert control over public health. on people's lives, especially in health crisis situations. During the pandemic, extreme measures such as confinement, mobility restrictions and mandatory vaccinations have been implemented, reflecting an intensified use of biopower. These interventions have been justified by the need to protect public health, but have also sparked debates about the ethics and limits of state control over individual bodies. Fear of contagion has been a powerful driver for the acceptance of these measures. The perception of risk has led many people to accept restrictions that, under normal circumstances, might be considered unacceptable. This phenomenon can be understood as a normalisation of biopower, where exceptional measures become everyday practices. The health crisis has generated a state of emergency that has allowed governments to extend their authority and oversight over the population, raising questions about the future of individual freedoms and human rights in crisis contexts.

The response to the pandemic has also revealed structural inequalities in access to health and health resources. The most vulnerable communities have been disproportionately affected by the virus and have had less access to treatment and vaccines. This highlights how biopower is not only exercised through health policies, but also through decisions that reflect economic and political interests. The management of the pandemic has shown that social control is not only a public health issue, but also a reflection of power dynamics in society.

The COVID-19 pandemic has prompted a debate on the ethics of biopower, and the decisions taken by governments during this crisis have been the subject of criticism and analysis from various philosophical and ethical perspectives. It is questioned whether the end justifies the means when it is is about protecting public health. This ethical dilemma is central to understanding how biopower has been exercised during the pandemic and what its implications are for the future of health policy and respect for individual rights.

Quarantine, containment and containment measures

During the pandemic, quarantines and mandatory confinement limited individual freedoms in the name of the common good, intensifying biopower as a tool to reduce the risk of contagion. According to Muñoz (2000), the decisions taken during pandemics may reflect both a commitment to public health and an exercise of biopower that may limit individual freedoms. During the COVID-19 pandemic, for example, many governments implemented drastic measures such as mandatory lockdowns and restrictions on public gatherings.

Western representative democracies have entered a deep crisis and the fight against the current COVID-19 pandemic has gradually led to the reduction or even suppression of elements traditionally linked to democratic life. The restriction of freedoms by confinement, the health pass, the obligation to wear masks in public spaces, the ever more intense blurring of the distinction between private and public life, the implementation of surveillance and control measures in the name of health security and security in general, are reaching a worrying threshold.

These phenomena are well known and identified as such, although the authorities applying the corresponding measures justify them by claiming that they are exceptional and temporary. "Afterwards everything will go back to the way it was", they promise. This is a way of paying tribute to those who denounce a serious disruption of democracy due to the protection apparatus used apparently only against the virus. Gigantism, the connivance of the different powers in international organisations, the refusal to consider other medical treatment tools and techniques, the hatred of those who propose other analyses and perspectives, open up the question, which seems inevitable, of whether the security pursued is not exclusively or really "health", but politically "security" (Mengue, 2022).

Information management and the management of public perception

Information management was crucial during the pandemic. State communication campaigns played a central role in guiding the behaviour of the population, managing the perception of risk, and promoting compliance with sanitary measures. Information management during the pandemic has been crucial in shaping public perception of COVID-19. Since the beginning of the outbreak, the overwhelming amount of information available has led to what is known as "infodemia", a term coined by the World Health Organisation to describe the rapid spread of erroneous or confusing information related to the virus. This has complicated efforts to effectively communicate preventive measures and the risks associated with infection. The lack of clarity in official messages has generated mistrust among the population towards health authorities. Effective information management requires adequate coordination between different actors involved in the health response. This includes governments, non-governmental organisations, the media and local communities. During the pandemic, some countries were able to establish effective platforms for sharing relevant and up-to-date information on COVID-19, which facilitated a more agile and effective response to the virus. However, others face significant challenges due to a lack of coordination or restrictive policies that limit the free flow of information. Public perception of risk has also been influenced by how information on COVID-19 is presented. Studies have shown that clear and transparent communication can increase trust in health authorities and encourage preventive behaviours among the population. On the other hand, contradictory or alarmist messages can lead to increased anxiety and resistance to follow health recommendations. Thus, proper information management is not only crucial to control the , but also to maintain an emotional balance in society.

CHAPTER 5

VACCINATION POLICIES AS AN EXPRESSION OF BIOPOWER

The history of vaccination and its social legitimisation

The history of vaccines can be traced back to ancient China, where writings from the XI refer to an early form of vaccination, known as "variolisation", which is the inoculation of smallpox pus to cause smallpox in an attenuated form and thus immunise the patient. This practice was not without risk, as a number of those vaccinated contracted smallpox in a severe form and eventually died. Variolisation was introduced in Europe (in Great Britain) in 1721. However, the first concrete smallpox vaccine was discovered by Jenner, an English country doctor who in 1796 carried out his experiment of immunisation with lymph from a form of cowpox (hence the name vaccine). He got the idea after hearing a farmer in his village claim that she would not get "bad smallpox" because she had already contracted "cowpox", since cowpox was a disease that produced a rash on the udder, and milkers could get this disease, which protected them from human smallpox. Jenner spent twenty years studying this phenomenon and how to develop a method of immunisation, which culminated in the creation of a new vaccine. of its vaccine. Subsequently, Louis Pasteur took a major step forward in the history of vaccines by demonstrating that administering a weakened or attenuated form of the infecting micro-organism produces a purer defence than introducing a germ that produces another disease similar to the one to be prevented. He developed vaccines against fowl cholera and anthrax, applying his discovery of attenuation. In 1885 he administered the rabies vaccine to a nine-year-old boy; this experiment was widely criticised because it involved the deliberate introduction of a deadly micro-organism into the human body, although it was a weakened micro-organism treated in a convenient way in his laboratory, and the success of the experiment was resounding. The late 19th century saw the development of killed microorganism vaccines against typhoid, cholera and plague, followed by the development of chemical inactivation of toxins, leading to the first toxoids: tetanus and diphtheria. The tuberculosis vaccine was developed in 1909. Other vaccines developed in this period were the yellow fever vaccine (1935) and the influenza A virus vaccine (1936).The golden age of vaccination began in 1949. After the polio vaccine, vaccines against measles, mumps and rubella were developed. The varicella vaccine was developed in the 1970s in Japan. Another live micro-organism vaccine introduced at this time was typhoid vaccine, and progress was also made in the development of inactivated vaccines against polio, rabies, Japanese encephalitis and hepatitis A.

Compulsory vaccination and individual rights

Evaccinations are one of the most important tools available to the state in the design of public policies for the fulfilment of its obligation to guarantee the right to health of the population. Its advantages lie in the eradication of infectious diseases and in ensuring equitable access of the population to this preventive instrument. Disadvantages permanent contraindications and temporary contraindications. The former include, by way of example, a severe allergic reaction (anaphylactic) to a previous dose of vaccine or to any of its components, and hypersensitivity or severe allergic reaction to any component of the vaccine. Among the latter, we mention cases of pregnancy, immunodeficiency and acute illness in which live virus vaccines have the potential to cause permanent injury or further aggravate the condition. clinical (Gázquez, 2019). According to the World Health Organisation (WHO), a vaccine is any preparation intended to generate immunity against a disease by stimulating the production of antibodies. It may be a suspension of killed or attenuated micro-organisms, or products or derivatives of micro-organisms. The most common method of administering vaccines is by injection, although some are administered by nasal or oral spray. Thus, vaccination is measure consisting of the administration of a preparation with the aim of preventing the occurrence of diseases, usually infectious, caused by the micro-organism against which the vaccine is administered; the vaccinated person is thus immunised against that particular micro-organism.

Compulsory vaccination raises debates about autonomy and individual rights and has been a controversial issue in many countries, with some arguing that it is necessary to protect the whole population, while others see the practice as an infringement of their personal freedoms. This ethical dilemma highlights how vaccination decisions can be viewed from different cultural and social perspectives. Furthermore, it is essential to consider how vaccine narratives have been influenced by anti-vaccine movements that question vaccine safety and efficacy. These movements reflect tensions between scientific knowledge and popular beliefs, which can further complicate the effective implementation of vaccine policies (Orenstein, 2019).

Incentives, restrictions and regulation of access

Fix vaccination is an essential component of public health, and its success depends to a large extent on the implementation of appropriate incentives to encourage participation. These incentives can be monetary, such as payments cash or gift cards, or non-cash incentives such as hygiene products or food. Evidence suggests that incentive programmes can significantly increase vaccination rates, as was observed during the COVID-19 pandemic, where an increase in intention to vaccinate was reported thanks to these incentives. However, it is crucial that these incentives are implemented in conjunction with other strategies that facilitate access to vaccines, such as free transportation and elimination of costs associated with vaccination.Restrictions also play an important role in access to vaccination. In many countries, laws exist that require certain population groups to receive specific vaccines as part of the National Immunisation Schedule. These regulations aim to ensure that all citizens have access to the immunisations necessary to protect public health. However, it is critical that these restrictions are applied fairly and equitably, and do not become barriers to those who face financial or logistical difficulties in accessing health services. Regulating access to vaccination involves establishing clear rules to ensure the availability and adequate supply of vaccines. Health authorities must ensure that vaccines are accessible and free to all citizens, eliminating any costs associated with their administration. In addition, it is essential that mechanisms are put in place to reach vulnerable and underserved communities, where access to health services may be limited. This includes conducting vaccination campaigns in community settings and providing clear information on the benefits and safety of vaccines.A critical aspect of regulating access is public confidence in vaccination programmes. Negative perceptions of vaccines can hinder efforts to increase immunisation rates. It is therefore vital that policymakers work to strengthen this trust transparent communication about the benefits and risks associated with vaccines. Continuing education and engagement with communities are key tools for addressing concerns and mitigating mistrust of health interventions. A comprehensive approach combining incentives, effective regulations and a strong communication strategy needs to be considered to maximise access to vaccination. Doing so will not only increase immunisation rates, but also contribute to building a more resilient and equitable health system. This approach should include constant evaluation of implemented policies and evidence-based adjustments to their effectiveness and public acceptance.

CHAPTER 6

ETHICS AND RIGHTS IN PUBLIC HEALTH MANAGEMENT

Individual vs. collective rights on health

Biopower applied to public health raises an essential question: how far can the state intervene in people's lives to protect collective health? This issue has generated important debates about the boundaries between individual rights and collective needs. The right to personal autonomy allows each individual to make decisions about his or her body and health, while the collective right to health protection implies that the state can impose certain regulations to avoid risks to the community. In situations such as pandemics, these tensions are particularly salient, as the safety of the population may require the limitation of some individual freedoms, such as mobility or privacy. Individual rights in health are closely linked to the principle of autonomy. This principle holds that each person has the right to make decisions about their own health, including decisions about medical treatment, access to health information and the choice to refuse certain interventions. Privacy is also a fundamental right within the healthcare context, ensuring that individuals' personal and medical information is not shared without their explicit consent. In many countries, data protection and human rights laws support individual autonomy as a basic pillar of the relationship between patients and health professionals. In addition, individual rights in health also encompass equal access to medical services. All people, regardless of their background, gender, or economic status, should have the opportunity to receive the care they need. However, while these rights are fundamental, they sometimes conflict with the collective welfare when, for example, an individual's decision puts public health at risk (as in the case of communicable diseases). Collective rights in health, on the other hand, relate to the protection of the well-being of the community as a . These rights seek to ensure that the entire population has access to adequate health services, irrespective of their personal or economic circumstances. At the collective level, priority is given to disease prevention, public health promotion and the creation of a healthy environment for the whole of society. Public health policies, especially those implemented in exceptional situations such as vaccination campaigns or health restrictions during pandemics, illustrate how collective rights can imply temporary restrictions on individual rights. In these contexts, the collective good may justify public health measures that temporarily limit individual freedoms, such as the isolation of infected persons or the obligation to vaccinate, in to protect the entire population from health risks. The main challenge lies in finding a balance between the two approaches. On the one hand, it is essential to protect individual rights to guarantee autonomy, privacy and personal dignity. On the other hand, collective rights must be promoted to ensure that public health policies, such as disease prevention strategies and equitable access to health care, are effectively implemented for the general welfare.

In situations of health crisis, such as a pandemic, the state may need to prioritise collective rights in order to protect the health of the population. This may involve imposing temporary restrictions on individual freedoms, such as border closures, mandatory quarantines or the imposition of social distancing measures. However, it is crucial that these measures are proportionate, based on scientific evidence and applied for a limited time to prevent them from becoming an exercise of unwarranted control over the citizenry.

In this framework, the concept of "conditional liberty" becomes relevant, as it suggests that the state has the ability to regulate individual liberty when it poses a potential risk to others. Examples of this approach include quarantines and mandatory vaccinations. However, in order for these measures not to be perceived as excessive control of citizens' lives, they must be well justified and transparently implemented. The clear justification of health policies and transparency in their implementation are key to preventing them from becoming a form of coercion or an abuse of power by the state. Such measures can conflict with the right to personal autonomy, especially when citizens feel that their freedom of choice is being infringed. A clear example is the use of vaccination certificates for access to certain places or activities, an effective strategy to control infection, but which can be interpreted as a form of indirect coercion for people to be vaccinated. In democratic societies, such measures require not only a clear and reasoned justification, but also a solid legal framework explaining the need to protect collective health. This helps to prevent biopower from being seen as an unbridled exercise of control over the citizenry, and instead is perceived as a legitimate mechanism for the common good.

Ethical Debates: Autonomy and Biopower in Public Health

The tension between biopower and individual autonomy poses an ethical dilemma of great relevance in the context of modern public health. Autonomy, a fundamental value in contemporary societies, is manifested in respect for informed consent to medical treatment and the freedom to refuse health interventions. However, the exercise of biopower can put this autonomy at risk when intervention measures are imposed that, although aimed at collective well-being, may be perceived as invasive or coercive, generating possible resistance. between citizens. An emblematic example of this complex relationship is compulsory vaccination, implemented in some societies as a strategy to protect the community through collective immunity. Although these health policies have proven to be effective in disease prevention, for some sectors they represent a violation of individual freedom, generating a rejection based on the defence of the right to decide about one's own body. During the COVID-19 pandemic, this conflict became particularly evident, as in several countries vaccination was established as a prerequisite for access to public spaces, giving rise to a profound ethical debate about self-determination and personal autonomy in the face of state control.

In their ethical analysis, Beauchamp and Childress (2013) stress the importance of the principles of autonomy and justice in health policy-making. Individual autonomy, they argue, can be compromised when the state resorts to restrictive measures in the name of the common good, forcing individuals to choose between their freedom of choice and the collective welfare. Public health ethics, then, faces the challenge of finding a balance between individual rights and shared responsibilities, preventing biopower from being perceived as an exercise of excessive and authoritarian control over the personal freedoms of citizens.

To mitigate this tension, it is essential that states adopt a transparent approach to communication and promote social dialogue around their health policies. Public health measures must be communicated in a clear and accessible manner, with an ethical rationale that justifies their necessity and promotes understanding and consensus. citizen. In this way, the state can implement policies that respect cultural diversity and individual preferences, and in turn, guarantee collective well-being, consolidating a framework of respect for individual autonomy within a society aware of its shared commitments and responsibilities.

The role of human rights organisations

Human rights organisations play an essential role in monitoring public health policies, ensuring that state interventions respect the dignity and fundamental rights of citizens. Their work is not limited to surveillance, but also seeks to protect those individuals who might be disproportionately affected by policies such as quarantines or compulsory vaccination, advocating for fairness and equity in treatment. In this way, these organisations act as a counterbalance to the power of the state, preventing health policies from drifting into authoritarian practices and ensuring that they are aligned with ethical and legal principles. During the COVID-19 pandemic, the role of these organisations became particularly relevant, issuing recommendations that measures of confinement, digital surveillance and contact tracing should respect fundamental rights, such as privacy and human dignity. This context highlighted the importance of keeping biopower under strict supervision to avoid abuses. While biopower can be effective in the management of health emergencies, its exercise must be controlled so that public policies do not degenerate into practices of excessive control over citizens. The intervention of human rights organisations seeks precisely to ensure this balance, recalling the need to protect collective well-being without compromising individual rights.

The work of these organisations is particularly crucial in times of crisis, when the risk of public health policies overstepping ethical and legal boundaries becomes more latent. In health emergencies, their role is to ensure that the state does not abuse surveillance or intervention tools which, although created to address the crisis, could become mechanisms of social control if they are not properly regulated. Human rights organisations, by intervening in these issues, act as guardians of individual freedom, keeping biopower within the limits of ethics and respect for rights.

In addition, these organisations advocate for the interests of the most vulnerable groups, promoting inclusive and equitable implementation of health policies. By speaking out on behalf of those who may be disproportionately affected by health policy measures, these organisations are also advocating on behalf of the most vulnerable groups. restrictive, these entities ensure that the implementation of public policies respects diversity and social justice. In this way, a human rights framework is strengthened in which collective well-being is pursued without compromising the dignity and autonomy of each individual.

CHAPTER 7

BIOPOWER AND NEW TECHNOLOGIES IN PUBLIC HEALTH

Digital surveillance and monitoring of health

In recent decades, the advance of digital technologies has opened new doors in the field of public health. Digital surveillance, understood as the collection and analysis of health data in real time, promises to substantially improve the quality of public health care. efficiency of health systems and people's quality of life. However, these technological advances also pose significant challenges in terms of privacy protection, information security and individual autonomy. One of the greatest achievements of digital surveillance is its ability to monitor people's health in real time, allowing health professionals to intervene more quickly and accurately. Devices such as glucose monitors, physical activity trackers or mobile apps allow patients and clinicians to access detailed information about individuals' well-being. This constant monitoring capability facilitates a more proactive approach to health, where early signs of disease can be identified and complications prevented before they become serious problems. In turn, the analysis of large volumes of data through algorithms and predictive models makes it possible to anticipate disease outbreaks, optimising public health resources. The collection of information on symptoms, behavioural patterns or even population mobility allows for the early detection of possible epidemics. In this sense, digital surveillance not only improves the response to health emergencies, but also contributes to a preventive health model, focused on identifying risks before they materialise into serious problems.

For example, during the COVID-19 pandemic, mobile applications were implemented to track contacts and report potential infections; however, this raised concerns about excessive state surveillance (Zuboff, 2019). Moreover, these technologies tend to be available primarily to those with access to digital devices and reliable internet; this can exacerbate existing inequalities between different socio-economic groups (Hargittai and Shaw, 2020). Another benefit of these technologies is the optimisation of medical resources. Electronic health records (EHRs) provide fast and efficient access to patients' medical records, facilitating coordination between different medical services and errors resulting from missing information. Moreover, by digitising data, health systems can make more efficient use of resources, allocating them according to real needs and demand.

Artificial intelligence and algorithms in healthcare management

Artificial intelligence (AI) and the use of algorithms have become key tools in modern healthcare systems. Their integration into healthcare management has radically transformed the way healthcare data is processed, analysed and used for decision-making. These advances make it possible not only to improve the efficiency of health systems, but also to optimise the response to emergencies and health crises, making artificial intelligence a central part of the state's biopower strategy. The concept of biopower, coined by the philosopher Michel Foucault, refers to the way in which governments exercise control over the bodies and lives of citizens, using various technological, political and administrative tools. In the context of health, artificial intelligence and algorithms function as extensions of this biopower, allowing the state not only to monitor public health, but also to predict, manage and, in some cases, directly influence people's behaviour to improve health outcomes. Artificial intelligence makes it possible to process and analyse large volumes of data, which would be humanly impossible to achieve in real time without the support of advanced algorithms. AI systems are able to identify complex patterns in data, make predictions about disease outbreaks, and optimise resource allocation in crisis situations. For example, during a pandemic, algorithms can help predict the spread of the virus, identify locations with the greatest need for medical care, and more efficiently distribute medical supplies. In this respect, AI plays a crucial role in prevention, crisis management and epidemic monitoring. By analysing large amounts of health data in real time, health authorities can detect early signs of infectious diseases and act more quickly and effectively. This not only improves emergency response capacity, but also optimises treatment and the distribution of resources such as medicines, protective equipment or vaccines. From a biopower perspective, artificial intelligence and algorithms offer the state a powerful health surveillance tool. The massive collection and analysis of health not only facilitates decision-making, but also allows governments to monitor in real time the health behaviour of the population. With this monitoring capability, governments can intervene proactively, setting public health policies, designing preventive campaigns or even modifying behaviours through incentives and penalties. A clear example of this is the use of algorithms to track population adherence to vaccination programmes or preventive treatments. By analysing patient health data, the state can identify risk groups, personalise interventions and design more effective policies. However, this monitoring power also raises concerns about privacy and social control. If not properly managed, AI technologies could be used to exert excessive control over individuals' lives, creating an environment in which people feel constantly monitored.

Risks and challenges of technology on biopower

The incorporation of technology in health systems and in the management of human life has opened new dimensions in the exercise of biopower, a concept that Michel Foucault defined as the way in which governments exercise control over the bodies and lives of individuals. Through various technological, political and administrative tools, biopower seeks to regulate and manage the health of populations, and, in many cases, to influence the behaviour and decisions of citizens. Advances in artificial intelligence, predictive algorithms, and massive data analysis are revolutionising healthcare management, but they also present inherent dangers that, if not properly addressed, can compromise fundamental principles such as privacy, autonomy and equity.

1. Surveillance and Social Control

One of the most obvious risks of technology applied to health management is the expansion of population surveillance. Advances in data collection through health devices, mobile apps and tracking systems allow governments to monitor in real time not only the health conditions of individuals, but also their behaviours and habits. While this can be useful for preventing disease outbreaks or improving resource management in health crises, it also creates a sense of control that can undermine personal autonomy.

Biopower is exercised, in part, through this capacity for mass surveillance. Without a clear regulatory framework to protect individual rights, the use of tracking technologies can become a form of social control. Instead of being a tool in the service of collective well-being, mass data collection could be used to manipulate behaviour or to impose health regulations that impinge excessively on personal freedom.

2. Loss of Privacy and Autonomy

The mass collection of health data poses serious risks to privacy and personal control. Sensitive data can be misused or exposed, affecting patient safety. In addition, the use of algorithms to impose behavioural patterns or penalising "risky" habits could reduce individual autonomy, making health decisions not entirely one's own, but determined by digital systems.

3. Discrimination and Algorithmic Bias

Health algorithms, while effective, can perpetuate pre-existing biases in the data they are trained on, which can lead to indirect discrimination against vulnerable groups, such as racial minorities or people with limited access to health care. Such algorithmic discrimination is not always obvious, but its effects are profound and can deepen existing inequalities in access to health care. For example, a diagnostic algorithm based on historical data may not take into account disparities in access to health care between different groups, leading to prioritisation of certain patients while disadvantaging others. This can result in people from marginalised communities, who do not have regular access to care, being undervalued, amplifying structural inequities and deepening the gap in access to care.

4. Digital Exclusion and Inequality of Access

The digital divide is a key challenge in the context of biopower and digital health. Although new technologies promise to improve access to and quality of healthcare, not all citizens have the same opportunities to benefit from them. Factors such as lack of access to electronic devices, reliable internet connections, or the availability of services in rural areas or low-income communities, place certain populations at a disadvantage compared to those who do have access to these technologies.

This digital exclusion not only limits access to the benefits of digital health, but also amplifies existing socio-economic inequalities. Instead of reducing disparities, technology can deepen gaps in the quality of care available, creating a new form of inequality in access to health. Thus, biopower is not only exercised through control over data, but also through control over the tools needed to access and fully participate in the digital health system.

5. Technological Dependency and the Dehumanisation of Care

Increasing reliance on health technologies can lead to the dehumanisation of healthcare. While algorithms improve efficiency, impersonal treatment and excessive automation can erode the trusting relationship between patients and healthcare professionals. The focus on data can reduce the patient to a numerical set, rather than considering their human and emotional context, affecting the quality of care and patient satisfaction.

It is therefore essential to strike a balance between the use of technology and preserving the human aspect of healthcare.

6. Concentration of Power and Data Privacy

Massive access to personal data by large technology companies poses risks of concentration of power and privatisation of health. These corporations can use data not only to improve public health, but also to generate commercial profits by selling personal information without proper consent. Without clear regulations on the management of this data, citizens are exposed to abuse of their private information by for-profit actors.

7. Ethical and Regulatory Challenges

Finally, one of the biggest challenges of digital biopower is the lack of ethical and legal regulation. Technology is advancing rapidly, but legislation often lags behind, leaving citizens vulnerable to abuse. The absence of clear regulatory frameworks on the use of personal data, transparency of algorithms and control over automated decisions can result in an environment where individuals' fundamental rights are compromised.

It is crucial that governments, institutions and health professionals work together to develop ethical and regulatory frameworks to ensure that technologies are used fairly, responsibly and for the benefit of society as a whole.

CHAPTER 8

FUTURE PERSPECTIVES IN PUBLIC HEALTH AND BIOPOWER

Public health in a globalised world

Globalisation has transformed all aspects of human life, including public health. In an interconnected world, advances in technology, international mobility and information exchange have given rise to new opportunities and, at the same , new challenges in health management. Diseases no longer recognise borders and, as global interactions increase, health issues extend beyond national boundaries, affecting both developed and countries alike. One of the greatest challenges in contemporary public health is the rapid spread of infectious diseases. In a world where people travel more than ever, epidemics can cross continents in a matter of days. Recent examples, such as the COVID-19 pandemic, the Ebola outbreak in Africa or the spread of the Zika virus in Latin America, have highlighted how vulnerable our societies are to global health threats. These crises reveal the need for effective international cooperation, as responses to health emergencies must be rapid and coordinated between nations. Despite significant advances in medicine and public health, inequalities access to health care remain a fundamental barrier. While some countries gain rapid access to vaccines, innovative treatments and cutting-edge medical technologies, many others face monumental difficulties in ensuring basic care for their populations. This disparity is not only a reflection of economic differences, but also a manifestation of global fractures that underscore the urgent need for an inclusive and equitable approach to addressing the world's health crises.

In this context, globalisation plays a crucial role. While it has generated advances in access to technologies and treatments in many parts of the world, it has also deepened inequalities. The social determinants of health, such as access to education, employment, social security, housing and the environment, have been profoundly affected by globalisation. influenced by global expansion. In many countries, economic disparities have widened, creating an even greater gap between those who can access quality health services and those who cannot. Poor living conditions, poverty, malnutrition and lack of access to clean water or basic health services remain some of the most persistent problems in global public health. One of the great promises that globalisation brings with it is access to new technologies in the field of health. Tools such as telemedicine, health information systems and the use of big data offer enormous opportunities to monitor, diagnose and treat diseases more efficiently, even in the most remote and underserved areas of the world. These advances have the potential to reduce inequalities by enabling easier and faster connection between patients and medical services, regardless of their geographical location. However, this promise is limited by inequalities in access to technology. In many regions, especially in countries, digital infrastructure remains inadequate. Lack of access to quality internet or appropriate devices limits the opportunities for individuals to benefit from these innovations. Instead of being an equaliser, technology can end up widening the gap, exacerbating pre-existing inequalities. Rural areas, the elderly or people in vulnerable situations are particularly affected, as they struggle the most to access these technological advances that could, in principle, improve their health and quality of life.

In this sense, globalisation has exacerbated inequalities, creating new obstacles for those already in vulnerable situations. While technology and scientific advances can be powerful tools, their impact is conditioned by the socio-economic barriers that continue to mark the reality of many populations. The opportunities offered by innovations must be accompanied by inclusive public policies that ensure that the benefits reach everyone, without leaving the most disadvantaged behind. Inequality in access to healthcare remains a critical challenge in the globalised world. To effectively address global health crises, it is necessary to implement an approach that considers not only technological innovations, but also the economic and social inequalities that condition access to health. Globalisation should be seen as an opportunity to narrow the gap rather than widen it, but only if the inequalities that mark access to health and technology are properly managed. The road to equitable global health is not only through access to medicines and technology, but also improved conditions, education and poverty reduction. Public policies must ensure that advances in health are accessible to all, regardless of their origin or resources. Health cannot be a luxury for the few, but a basic right for all human beings.

Biopower policies in the context of climate change

Elimate change stands as one of the greatest public health challenges of future, and calls for an expansion of biopower policies to address its multiple and profound consequences. Alterations in climate and Environmental conditions are leading to an increase in the incidence of vector-borne diseases, such as dengue and malaria, which thrive in increasingly hot and humid environments. In addition, phenomena such as extreme heat waves, water scarcity and population displacement due to extreme weather events additional burdens on health systems and generate new risks that the state must manage. In the face of these challenges, it is essential to develop adaptation and mitigation policies that protect the health of communities in an environment increasingly vulnerable to climate change. The fight against climate change also raises the need to change certain collective behavioural patterns, particularly in terms of resource consumption and pollution practices. Biopower, in this context, can play a key role in environmental awareness and education, guiding citizens towards more sustainable habits that minimise environmental impact while protecting public health. The State, in this sense, has the potential to regulate and encourage practices that favour a responsible use of natural resources and contribute to reducing the harmful effects of climate change. In this way, it promotes a cultural change that seeks to integrate sustainability into people's daily decisions, laying the foundations for a more harmonious coexistence with the natural environment.To adequately respond to the health challenges posed by climate change, it is crucial to anticipate the impact of these dynamics on future public health policies. According to Kickbusch (2016) this approach requires not only the implementation of traditional health measures, but also the exploration of alternative models that incorporate social equity and community inclusion as fundamental principles. policies could ensure that state interventions respond to the needs of the most vulnerable populations and promote equitable access to resources and health care. In addition, the complexity of health and climate change issues demands an intersectoral approach that integrates diverse perspectives, fostering dialogues between sectors such as environment, economy and infrastructure. Only through collaboration and understanding of these multiple angles will it be possible to develop public health that not only respond to current challenges, but also anticipate emerging issues arising from climate change. This holistic approach allows public health policies to go beyond tackling isolated symptoms and address the underlying causes and strengthen the resilience of communities in the face of changes that are already transforming the planet.

The future of biopower in ethics and governance

The future of biopower in public health will largely depend on its ability to address ethical challenges and adapt to the growing demands for transparency, fairness and equity in health governance. The increasing integration of digital technologies, constant health monitoring and the use of automated systems offer great opportunities to improve public health. However, they also pose serious risks related to privacy, autonomy and social justice. For biopower to be effective in protecting collective health, it is crucial to set clear limits on its implementation and ensure independent oversight by external bodies and civil society. Public health governance must be based on fundamental principles such as transparency, citizen participation and equity, enabling people to understand and have a say in the policies that affect their lives and health. In an interdependent world, biopower must evolve into a tool that not only protects health, but also respects and promotes human rights and social justice. This evolution will ensure the legitimacy of biopower in democratic societies and the effectiveness of its policies in combating health inequalities.

As technological systems play a more crucial role in health management, ethical dilemmas arise that require in-depth debate. Decisions about people's health should not only be technical or administrative; they should be based on ethical principles that respect autonomy, privacy, justice and accountability. Technological advances, such as artificial intelligence in diagnosis and digital health, can offer benefits, but they must be implemented with an approach that preserves individual rights and does not become tools of control. Ethical reflection on the power that the actors involved (governments, health institutions and technology companies) have over the lives and well-being of citizens is essential to ensure that biopower used fairly and responsibly. Central to the biopower of the future will be the construction of global health governance, in which countries work together to create an inclusive and equitable health system. This global collaboration should seek to reduce inequalities in access to health services, promoting equitable access to technologies and treatments for all sectors of the population, regardless of their geographic location or socio-economic status. Technology and innovation in health should be tools at the service of human well-being, not means to exercise control or surveillance over people. Furthermore, health technologies must be designed and regulated under an ethical framework that prioritises the rights and needs of individuals. This approach implies an ethics of care, in which technological interventions are implemented with a critical awareness of their ethical, social and political implications. Biopower must be a driving force for improving the quality of life, but without sacrificing people's autonomy and dignity. If properly managed, these tools can contribute to the creation of a more humanised health , where health protection and collective well-being do not become a form of oppression, but a means to strengthen the health of the entire population.

REFERENCES

Assembly National Assembly at National Assembly of Nicaragua. (2007). Law General   de Health. http://legislacion.asamblea.gob.ni/Normaweb.nsf/($All)/FF82EA58EC7C712E06 257 0A1005810E1

Agamben, G. (2024). Homo sacer. Sovereign power and bare life. Adriana Hidalgo Editora. https://books.google.es/books?hl=es&lr=&id=T9oJEQAAQBAJ&oi=fnd&pg=PT 6&dq=related:CtB9NTImN9gJ:scholar.google.com/&ots=AeQI6J4ci2&sig=2q83 ybOFMI 2-w_gp7V7kk87GAFo

Beauchamp, T., & Childress, J. (2013). Principles of biomedical ethics (7th ed.). Oxford University Press. https://www.unprofesor.com/filosofia/principios-de-etica- biomedicine-of-beauchamp-and-childress-summary-and-conclusions/

Crawford, R. (2006). Health as a meaningful social practice: The role of the state in health promotion and the management of risk in the United States and Canada since the mid-20th century. Social Science & Medicine, 62(2), 293-302. https://journals.sagepub.com/doi/abs/10.1177/1363459306067310

Campos Fernández, E. (2010). Historia de la sexualidad 1: La voluntad del saber de Michel Foucault. Sapiens, 11(1), 231-233. http://ve.scielo.org/scielo.php?script=sci_arttext&pid=S1317-58152010000100014Esposito, R. (2012). Immunity, community, biopolitics. The Towers of Lucca: international journal of philosophy politics, 1(1), 101-114. https://dialnet.unirioja.es/servlet/articulo?codigo=4588647

Ertl, H. C., Zaia, J., Rosenberg, S. A., June, C. H., Dotti, G., Kahn, J.& Strome, S. E. (2011). Considerations for the clinical application of chimeric antigen receptor T cells: observations from a recombinant DNA Advisory Committee Symposium held June 15, 2010. Cancer research, 71(9), 3175-3181. https://aacrjournals.org/cancerres/article-abstract/71/9/3175/575477

Foucault, M. (2009). Birth of biopolitics: course at the Collège de France (1978-1979) (Vol. 283). Editions Akal. https://books.google.es/books?hl=es&lr=&id=tvgjUSb1WG4C&oi=fnd&pg=PA4&dq=The+birth+of+biopoli%C3%ADtica.+Fund+of+Econ%C3%B3mica.&ots=9_-36jfwud&sig=rsGl5v1NspnWI6ehJWdkWDQ1AY4

García, A., & González, M. (2015). Education and biopolitics: A critical analysis. Revista de Estudios Social, 54, 110-123. https://revistas.unal.edu.co/index.php/index/login?source=%2Findex.php%2Festudios-sociales%2Farticle%2Fview%2F48705

Gázquez, M. Y. (2019). Law, health and public policy. Vaccination. Positions for and against. Journal Derecho y Salud, 3(3), 62-75. https://revistas.ubp.edu.ar/index.php/rdys/article/view/59

González, F. M., & Jiménez, M. C. (2018). Hanlon's method, a methodological tool for prioritizing health needs and problems. An operational perspective for health diagnosis. Vertientes. Revista especializada en ciencias de la salud, 21(1-2), 42-49. https://revistas.unam.mx/index.php/vertientes/article/view/72839

Hargittai, E., & Shaw, A. (2020). Mind the gap: The interplay between digital inequality and health disparities during COVID-19 pandemic in the U.S. Health Affairs, 39(10), Article1685. https://www.healthaffairs.org/doi/full/10.1377/hlthaff.2020.00897

Kickbusch, I., Allen, L., & Franz, C. (2016). The commercial determinants of health. The Lancet Global Health. https://www.thelancet.com/journals/langlo/article/PIIS2214-109X(16)30217-0/fulltext.

López-Acuña, D., Muñoz, F., & Halverson, P. (2014). The essential functions of public health: An emerging theme in sector reforms. Rev Panam Salud Pública, 8(1/2), 1-12. https://www.scielosp.org/pdf/rpsp/v8n1-2/3012.pdf

Muñoz, F., López-Acuña, D., Halverson, P., et al. (2000). The essential functions of public health: An emerging theme in health sector reforms. Rev

Panam Salud Pública, 8(1/2), 1-12. https://www.scielosp.org/pdf/rpsp/v8n1-2/3012.pdf

Mengue, P. (2022). Biopower in the age of the pandemic. Revista latinoamericana de filosofía, 48(2), 1-10. http://www.scielo.org.ar/scielo.php?pid=S1852-73532022000200001&script=sci_arttext

Orenstein, W.A., et al. (2019). The role of vaccination in preventing disease outbreaks in children. Pediatrics, 144(2), Article e20193473. https://ve.scielo.org/scielo.php?script=sci_arttext&pid=S1316-71382012000100006.

WHO. (1946). Constitution of the Organisation World Organisation of the https://www.who.int/es/about/governance/constitution https://www.who.int/es/about/governance/constitution https://www.scielosp.org/article/ssm/content/raw/?resource_ssm_path=/media/assets/r bepid/v16n1/1415-790X-rbepid-16-01-0003.pdf

Oñate, B., Vilahur, G., Ferrer-Lorente, R., Ybarra, J., Díez-Caballero, A., Ballesta-López, C., & Badimon, L. (2012). The subcutaneous adipose tissue reservoir of functionally active stem cells is reduced in obese patients. The FASEB Journal, 26(10), 4327-4336.

https://faseb.onlinelibrary.wiley.com/doi/abs/10.1096/fj.12-207217

Rodríguez Milord, D. (2014). Public health surveillance, an instrument for the efficiency and sustainability of the Cuban health system. Revista Cubana de Higiene y Epidemiología, 52(3), 286-289.http://scielo.sld.cu/scielo.php?pid=S1561-30032014000300001&script=sci_arttext&tlng=pt

Zuboff, S. (2019, January). Surveillance capitalism and the challenge of collective action. In New labor forum (Vol. 28, No. 1, pp. 10-29). Sage CA: Los Angeles, CA: SAGE Publications. https://journals.sagepub.com/doi/abs/10.1177/1095796018819461